Table of Contents

Mexican Breakfast Scramble

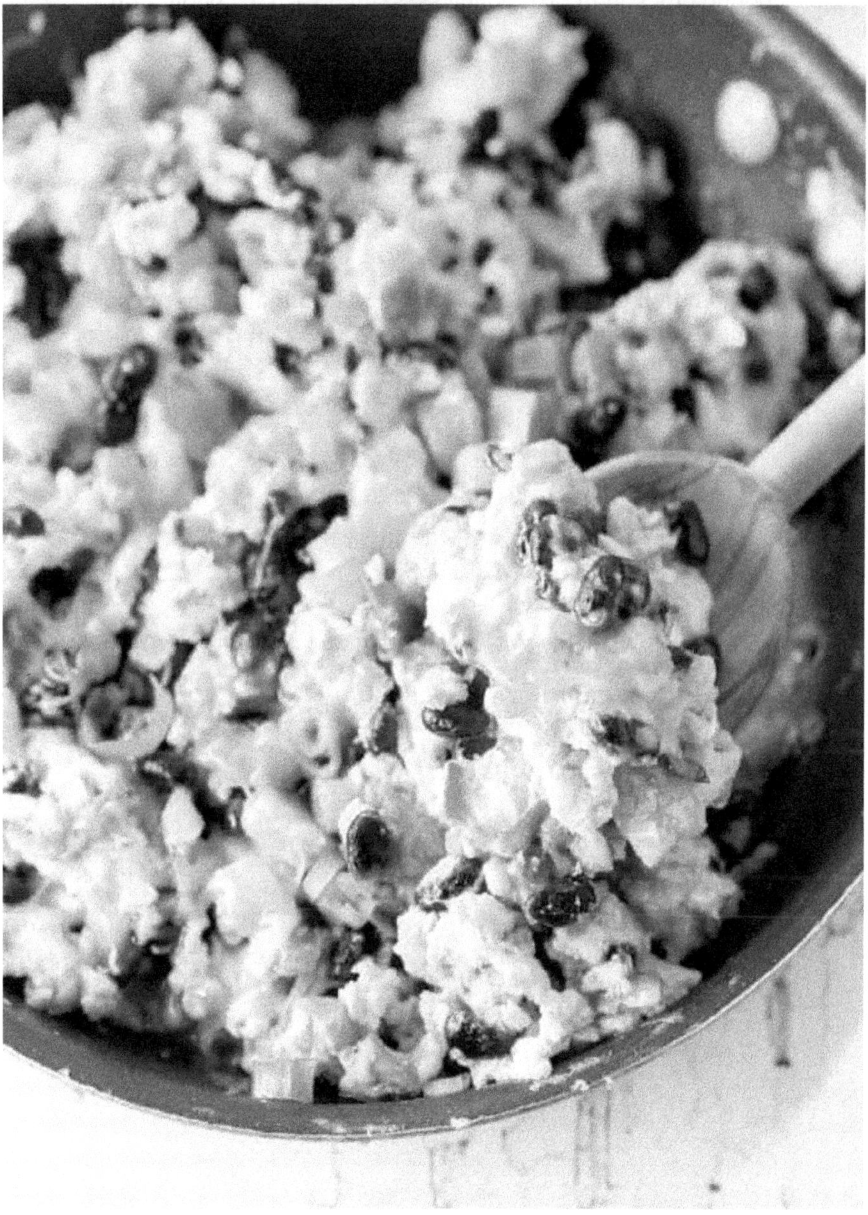

Prep Time

Total Time: 30 minutes Serves: 2

Ingredients:

1 tbsp. coconut oil for cooking chicken

¾ pound chicken breast, boneless, skinless 1 tsp. coconut oil

4 large eggs

½ tsp. cumin

½ tsp. chili powder

¼ tsp. sea salt 1 tbsp. water

¼ medium onion, red diced

1 medium bell pepper, green diced 1 medium jalapeno pepper, diced 1 medium tomato, diced

¼ cup cilantro, fresh chopped

Directions:

1. Heat a large sauté pan over medium-high heat and add coconut oil. Season chicken breasts with seas salt and pepper if desired and sauté for 10-15 minutes, turning once or twice until fully cooked. Chop into bite-size pieces.
2. Heat coconut oil in a medium skillet over medium-high heat.
3. Meanwhile, break eggs into a small bowl. Add cumin, chili power, sea salt, and water. Scramble with a fork until fully combined.
4. Add onions, bell peppers, and jalapeno to the hot skillet. Sauté 3-5 minutes, or until slightly softened.
5. Add eggs and pre-cooked chicken, and cook while continuously stirring until eggs are light and fluffy.
6. Remove from heat. Stir tomatoes, and top with fresh cilantro to serve.

Salmon Scrambled Eggs

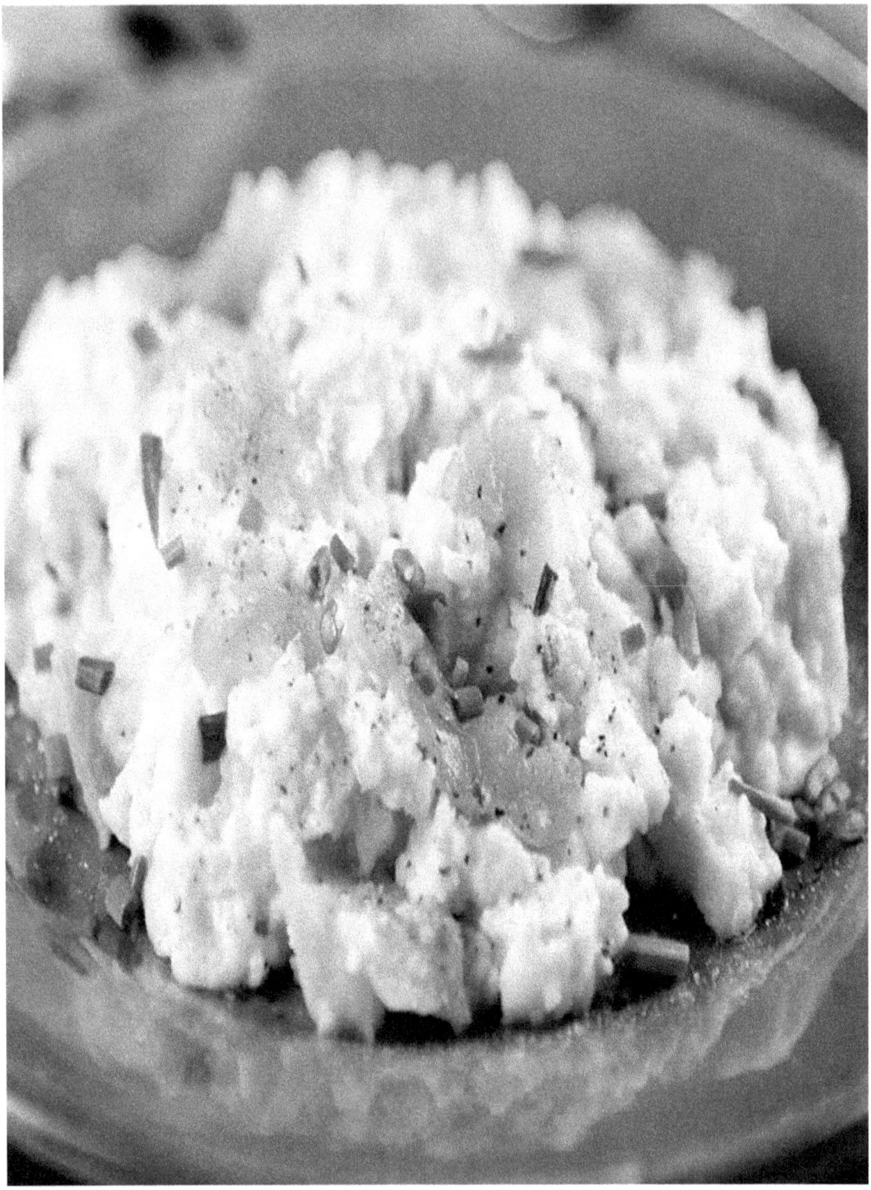

Prep Time

Total Time: 15 minutes Serves: 2

Ingredients:

1 tsp. coconut oil 4 large eggs

1 tbsp. water

4-ounce salmon smoked, cut into small pieces

½ medium avocado

¼ tsp. black pepper freshly ground 1 tbsp. chives minced

Directions:

1. Heat a medium skillet over medium heat. Add coconut oil to pan.
2. Meanwhile, crack eggs into a small bowl. Add water and scramble with a fork.
3. Add eggs to hot skillet, with salmon. Stir continuously , cook eggs until soft and fluffy.
4. Remove from heat. Top with black peppers, avocado, and chives.

Almond Butter, Bananas & Coconut

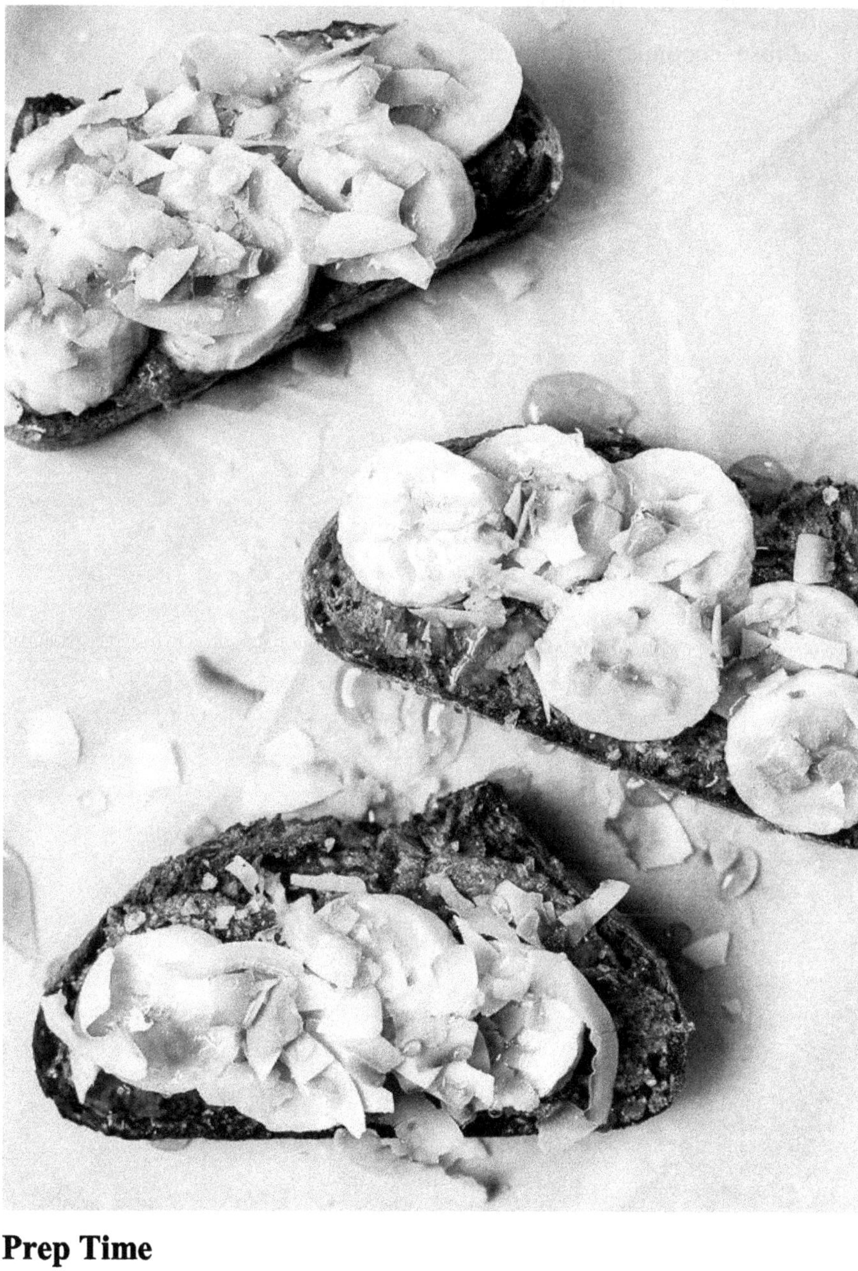

Prep Time

Total Time: 5 minutes Serves: 2

Ingredients:

1 large banana

2 tbsp. almond butter

2 tbsp. coconut milk, full fat

Directions:

1. Slice banana and divide into small bowls.
2. Top each banana half with half of the almond butter and coconut milk.

Eggs with Bacon & Veggies

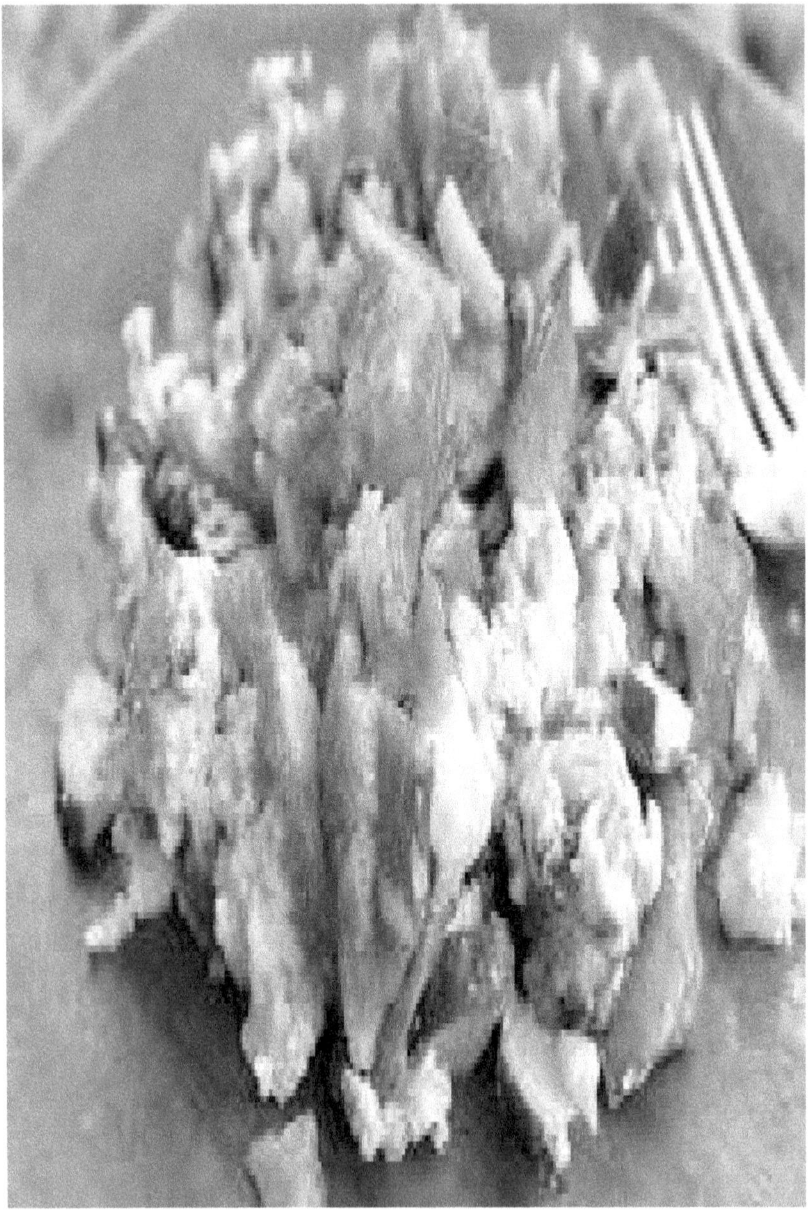

Prep Time

Total Time: 20 minutes Serves: 2

Ingredients:

4 slices bacon

4 large eggs

1 medium zucchini diced

1 medium garlic clove minced 1 medium tomato diced

1 cup spinach

Directions:

1. Cook bacon, remove from pan and reserve 1 tbsp. of the bacon drippings in the pan.
2. Meanwhile, wash and chop the veggies.
3. Over medium-high heat, add the zucchini, garlic and tomato to the pan with the remaining bacon drippings. Sauté until just before tender
4. While cooking, beat eggs in a small bowl. Set aside.
5. Crumble cooked bacon and set aside.
6. When the vegetables are almost done, add the beaten eggs and crumble bacon to the pan, along with the fresh spinach. Turn heat to medium-low and cook until the eggs are fluffy and firm.
7. Season with freshly ground black pepper and sea salt, if desired.

Zucchini Fritters

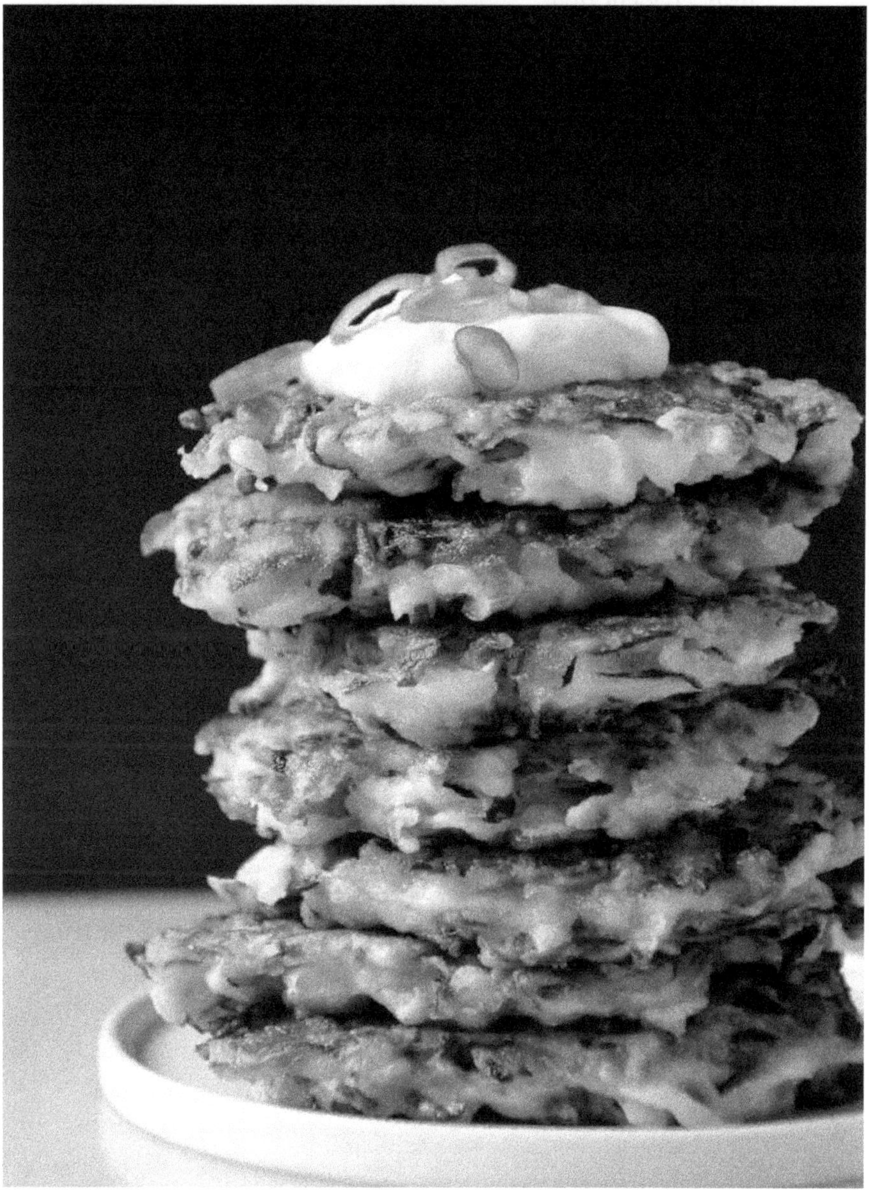

Prep Time

Total Time: 20 minutes Serves: 2

Ingredients:

2 medium zucchini shredded 3 large eggs

1 tbsp. coconut flour

½ tsp. sea salt

¼ tsp. black pepper, fresh ground 2 tbsp. coconut oil

Directions:

1. Shred zucchini by hand or in a food processor and set aside.
2. In a large bowl, beat eggs together.
3. Sift coconut flour into eggs and beat together
4. Mix shredded zucchini, sea salt and freshly ground black pepper together, and combine with egg mixture.
5. Meanwhile, set a large cast iron skillet over medium-low heat. When hot, add coconut oil to bottom of the pan.
6. Spoon the mixture into the pan in desired sized fritters.
7. Serve warm or at room temp.
8. Optionally: add other spices or fresh herbs and serve.

Applesauce, Almonds & Ham

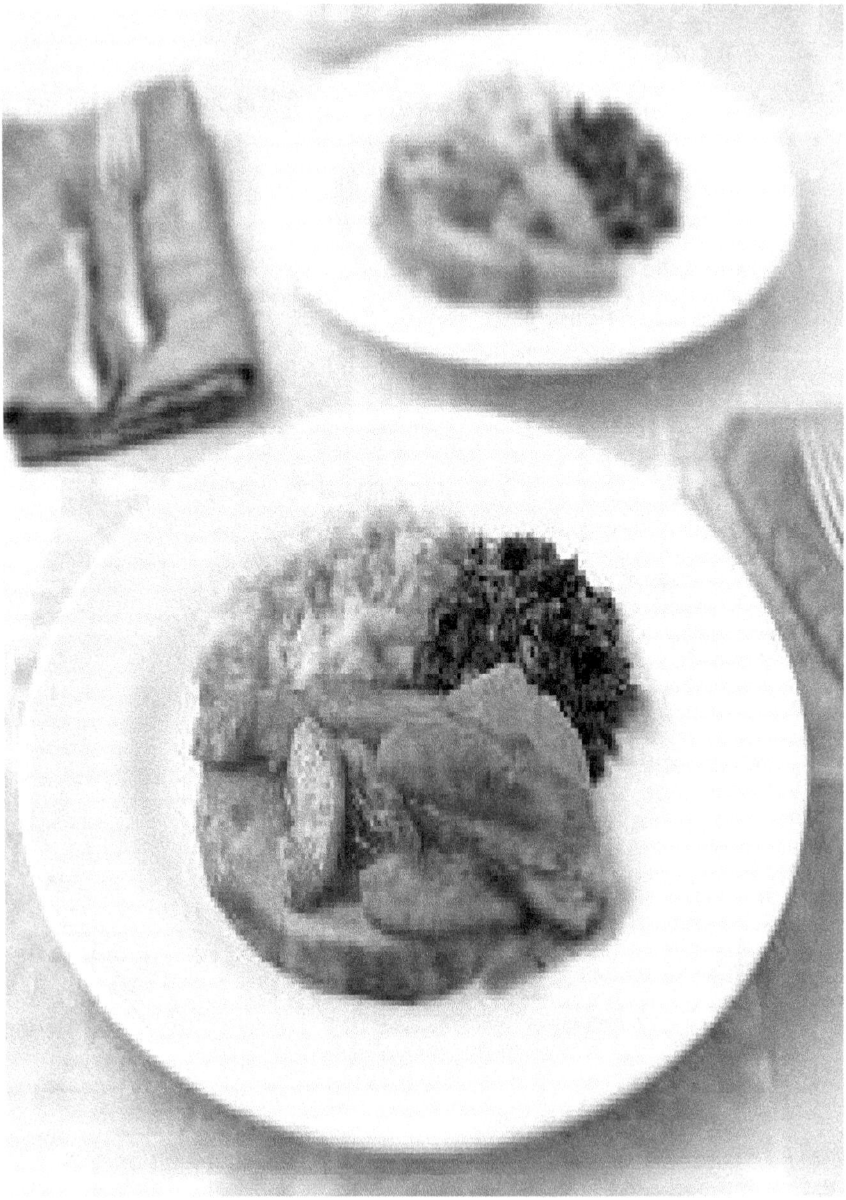

Prep Time

Total Time: 10 minutes Serves: 2

Ingredients:

¾ pounds' ham

2 cups applesauce, unsweetened (natural)

¾ cups almond

Directions:

1. Slice the ham and warm in a skillet on the stove.
2. Serve alongside applesauce and almonds.

Almond Banana Pancakes

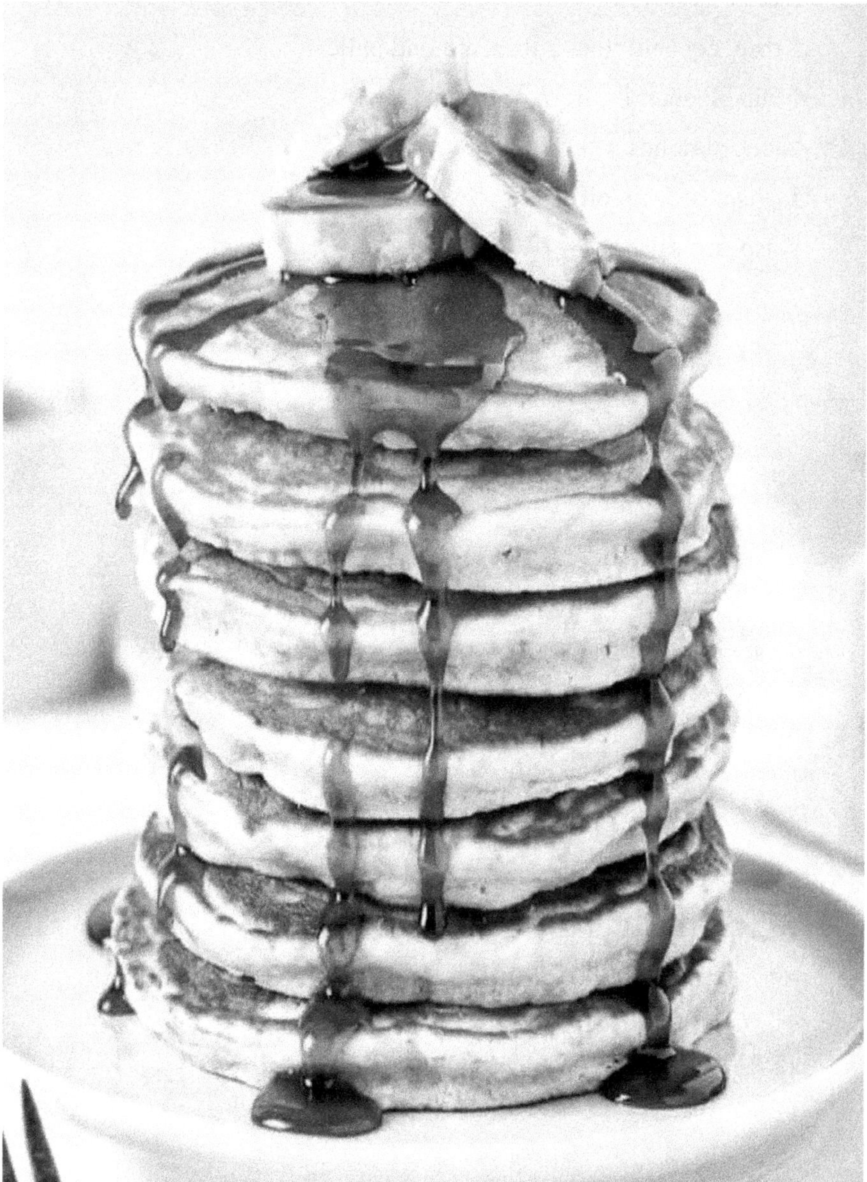

Prep Time

Total Time: 25 minutes Serves: 2

Ingredients:

2 medium bananas

2 large eggs

1 tbsp. coconut flour 2 tbsp. almond butter

1 cup blueberries, fresh or frozen

¼ cup almonds

1 tsp. coconut oil

¼ tsp. sea salt

Directions:

1. Mash bananas in a bowl
2. Add the eggs, coconut flour, almond butter, blueberries, and nuts and salt, and whisk until well blended.
3. Heat a large non-stick skillet over medium heat along with a small pat of coconut oil.
4. Pour small discs of batter onto the hot pan. They'll be easier to flip if you keep them from the edges of the pan.
5. Flip when batter loses its tackiness around the edges
6. Cook other side slowly over medium heat until fully cooked.
7. Reapply oil to the pan after each round of pancakes.

Oat-less Oatmeal

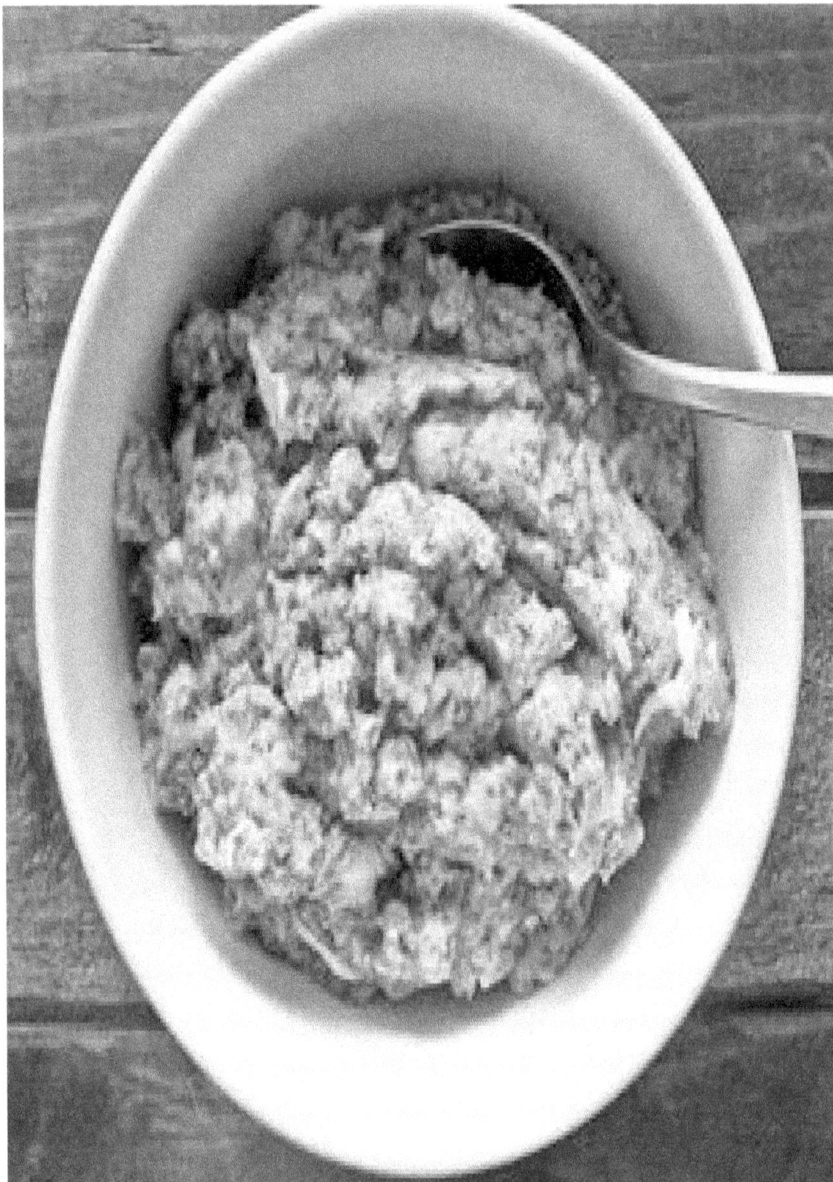

Prep Time

Total Time: 15 minutes Serves: 2 minutes

Ingredients:

¼ cup walnuts

¼ cup pecans

2 tbsp. ground flax seeds

½ tsp. cinnamon

¼ tsp. ground nutmeg

¼ tsp. ground ginger 1 tbsp. almond butter

1 medium mashed banana 3 large eggs

¼ cup almond milk, unsweetened 2 tbsp. pumpkin seeds

½ cup fresh berries (optional)

Directions:

1. Add walnuts, pecans, flax seed and spices to a food processor and pulse mixture to a coarse grain. Set aside.
2. Whisk together eggs and almond milk until the consistency thickens and becomes a loose custard.
3. Thoroughly blend the mashed banana and almond butter together and add it to the custard, mixing well.
4. Stir in the coarse nut mixture.
5. In a medium saucepan, warm the mixture on the stove until the Oat-less Oatmeal reaches the desired consistency and the whisked eggs look firm as though cooked. This should only take about 5 minutes.
6. Sprinkle pumpkin seeds and berries on top. Add more almond milk if desired.

Tapioca Crepes

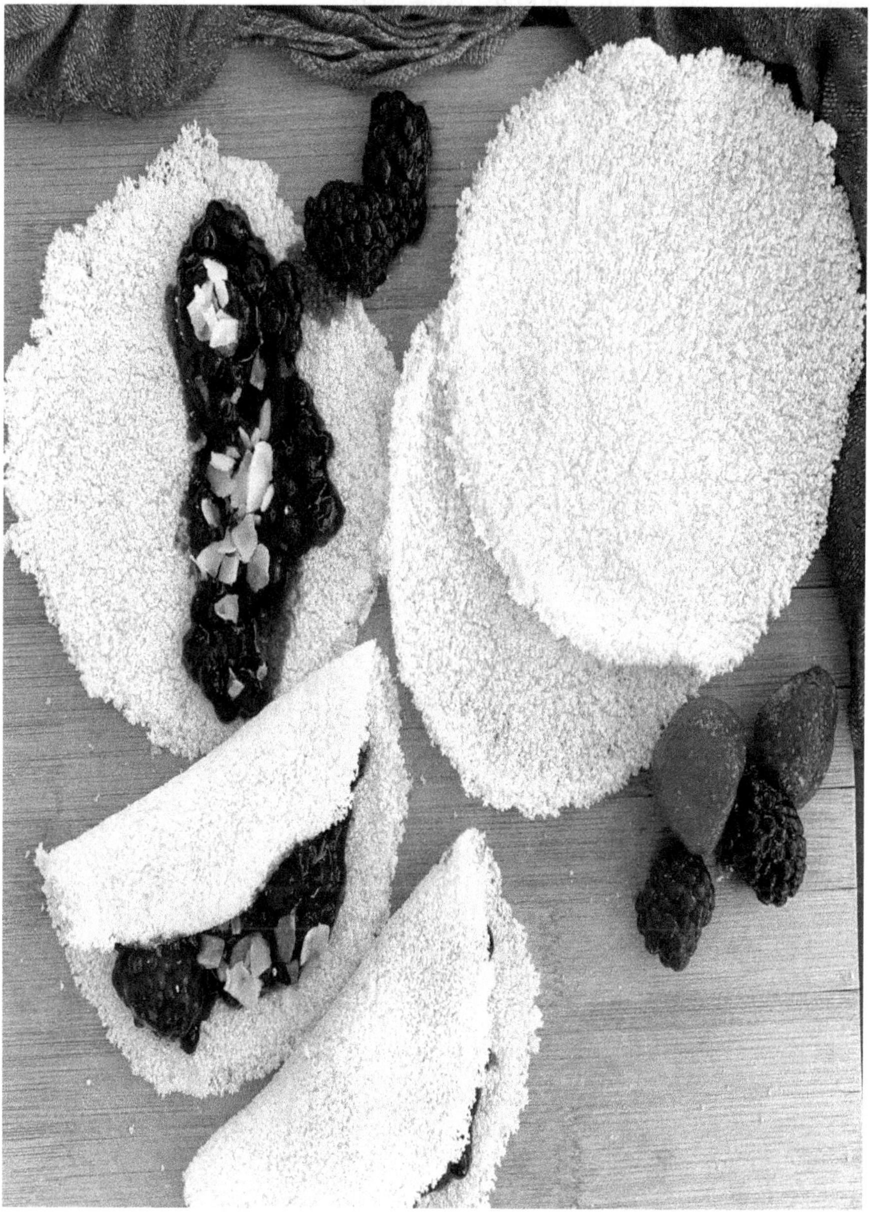

Prep Time

Total Time: 25 minutes Serves: 2

Ingredients:

1 cup tapioca flour

1 cup coconut milk, full fat 1 large egg

¼ tsp. sea salt

1 topping of choice

Directions:

1. Combine all the ingredients in a medium bowl and mix completely.
2. Heat a non-stick skillet over medium heat.
3. When hot, pour in about 1/3 cup of the mixture and tilt the pan in all directions to spread out batter to desired thickness.
4. Cook both sides until very lightly browned.
5. Top with desired ingredients and serve warm or cold.

Summer Frittata

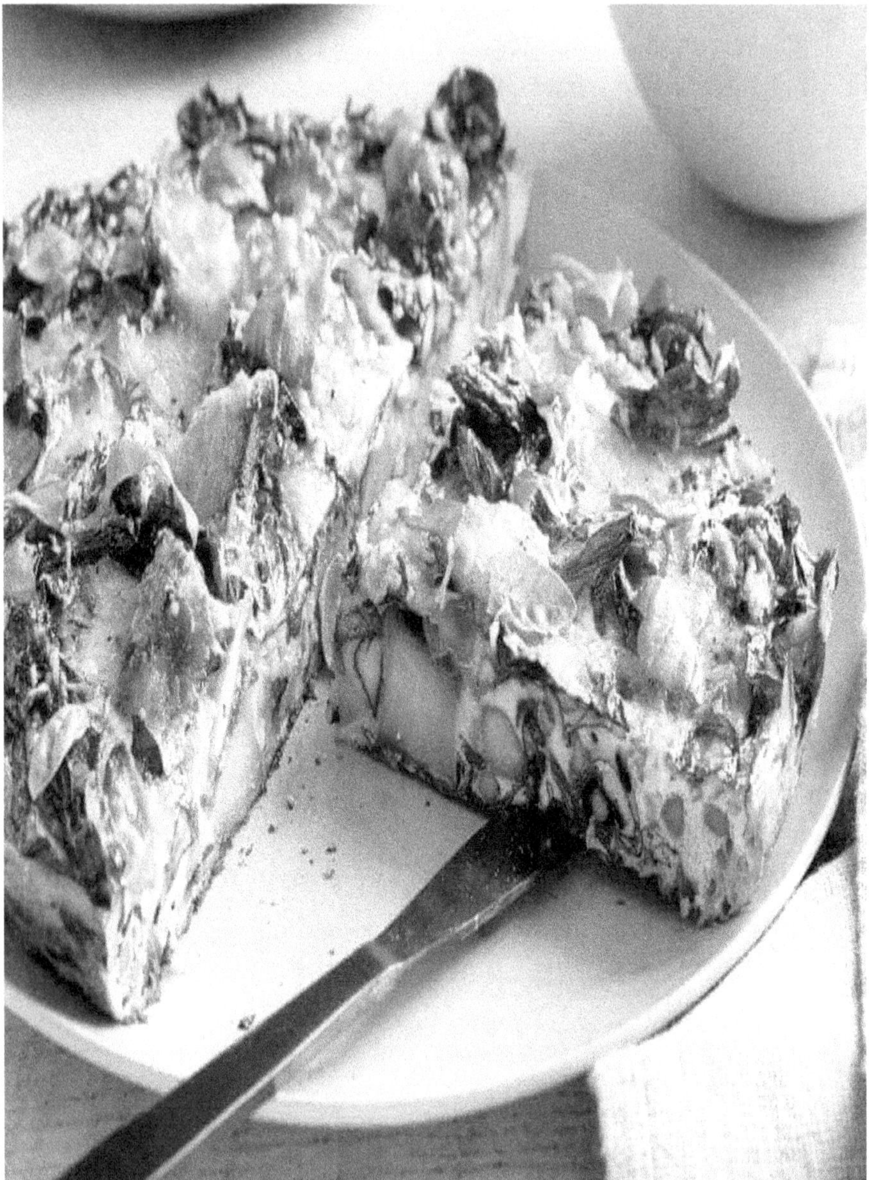

Prep Time

Total Time: 35 minutes Serves: 4

Ingredients:

1 ½ tbsp. coconut oil

1 medium zucchini diced

½ medium bell pepper, red sliced

½ red diced onion 1 tbsp. thyme

½ tsp. sea salt divided

¼ tsp. black pepper, divided

2 medium garlic cloves minced

1 medium tomato seeded and chopped 9 large eggs

Directions:

1. Heat coconut oil in a 10-inch oven-proof skillet over medium heat. When hot, add zucchini, pepper, onion, thyme, garlic and half of the sea salt and pepper.
2. Cover and cook until veggies are tender.
3. Stir in tomato. Cook, uncovered, for 5 minutes more or until liquid evaporates.
4. Combine eggs and remaining sea salt and pepper and whisk until frothy
5. Pour eggs over veggie mixture and stir gently. Cover, reduce heat and cook 15 minutes.
6. Meanwhile, preheat broiler to low Finish frittata with 3 minutes under the broiler.
7. Inver onto a plate, slice and serve warm or cold.

Guacamole Devils

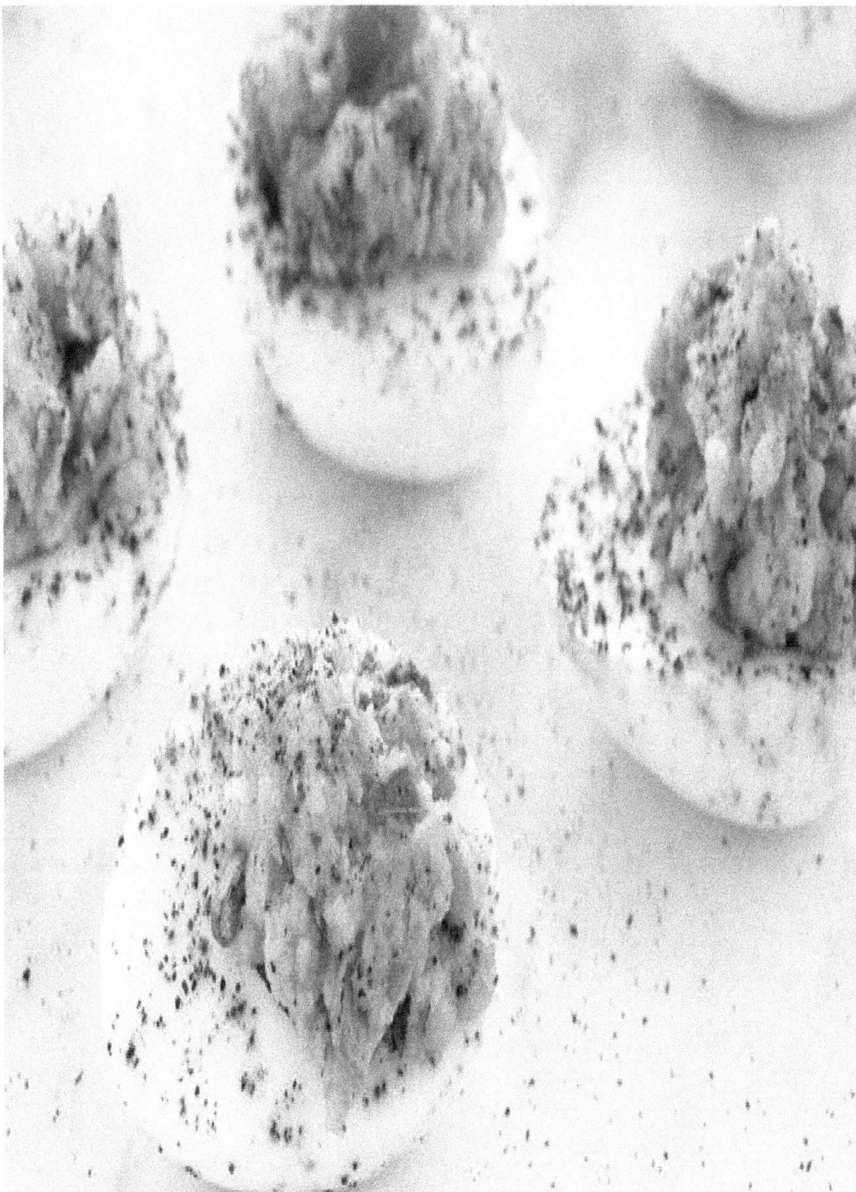

Prep Time

Total Time: 25 minutes Serves: 2

Ingredients:

4 large eggs hard-boiled 1 medium avocado

2 tsp. hot pepper sauce 1 tsp. lemon juice

¼ tsp. sea salt

¼ tsp. black pepper, fresh ground

Directions:

1. Peel hard-boiled eggs and cut in half length-wise. Spoon out yolks into a small bowl.
2. Mash yolks with avocado, hot sauce and lemon juice. Season with sea salt and freshly ground black pepper to taste.
3. Refill egg whites with the yolk mixture.

Eggies & Veggies

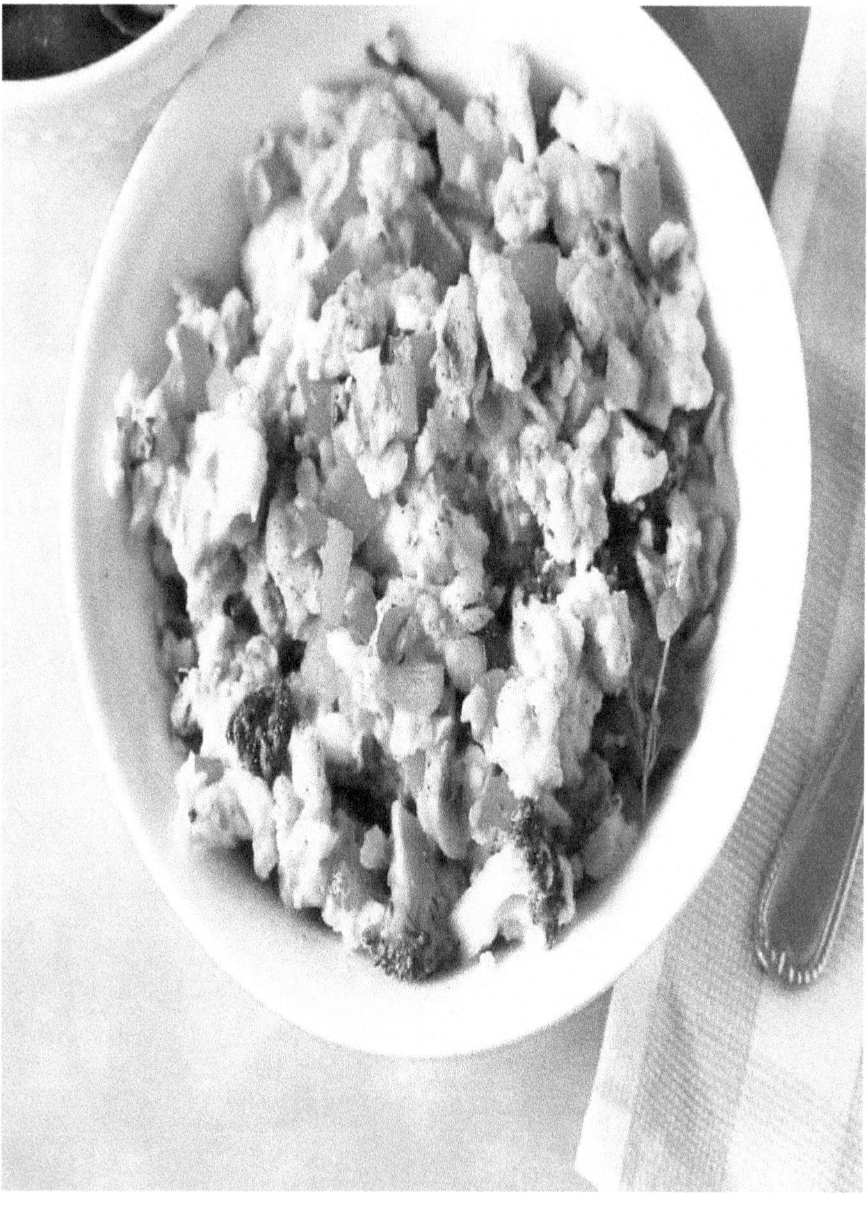

Prep Time

Total Time: 30 minutes Serves: 2

Ingredients:

4 slices bacon (reserve 1 tbsp. bacon grease)

¼ medium diced yellow onion 6 large chopped kale leaves

1 medium minced garlic clove 4 large eggs

1 medium sliced avocado

Directions:

1. Cook bacon. Remove from pan and put on paper towel to absorb extra oil. Crumble bacon when cool, and set aside.
2. Drain pan of all but a coating of bacon grease.
3. Sauté onion in bacon grease until slightly translucent. Add garlic and kale to pan and continue to cook until tender. Remove to two plates.
4. With the pan still hot, cook the eggs over easy in the leftover juices of the sauté
5. When the eggs are cooked, layer them on top of the vegetables.
6. Top with the sliced avocado and crumbled bacon.

Paleo PP&J

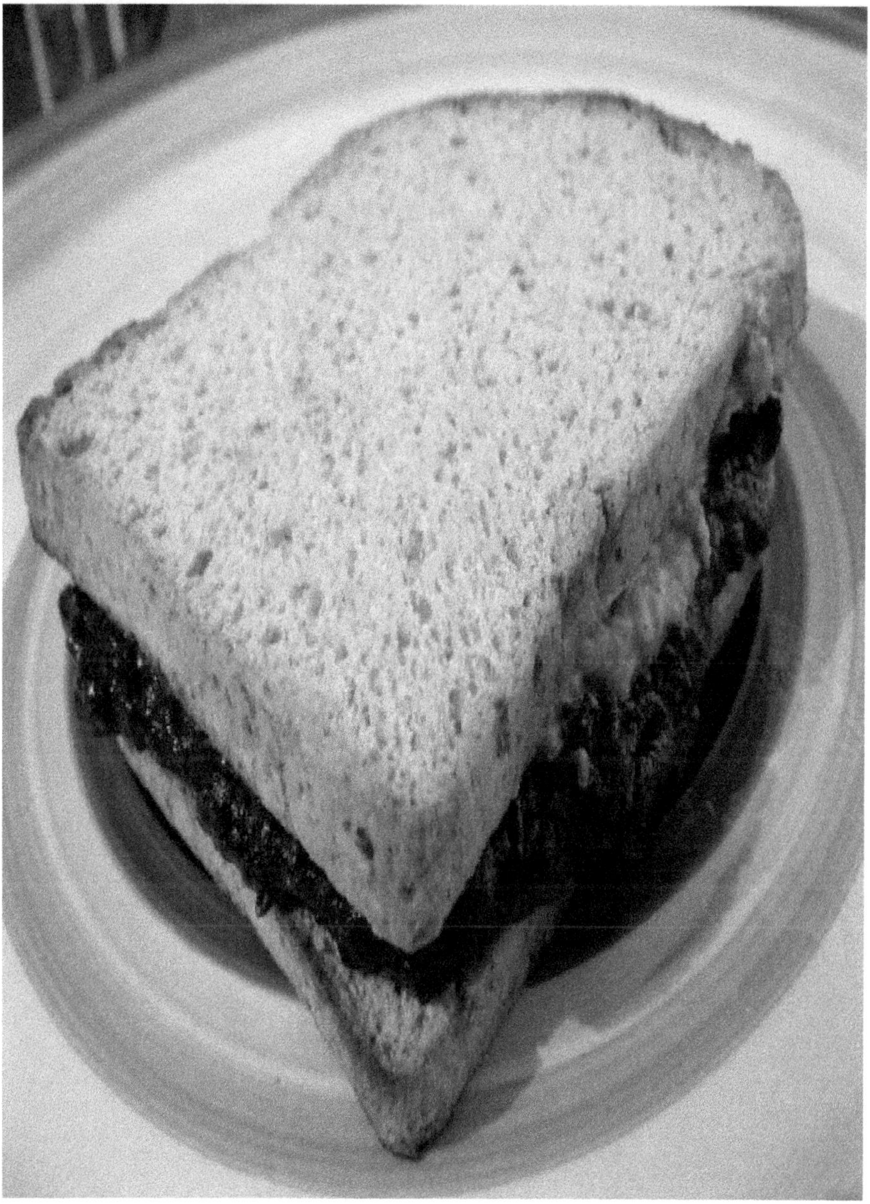

Prep Time

Total Time: 5 minutes Serves: 2

Ingredients:

1 cup fresh or frozen berries 4 tbsps. almond butter

Directions:

1. Divide the berries into serving bowls.
2. Add 2 tbsps. Almond butter to each bowl and mix.

Shrimp Omelet with Avocado

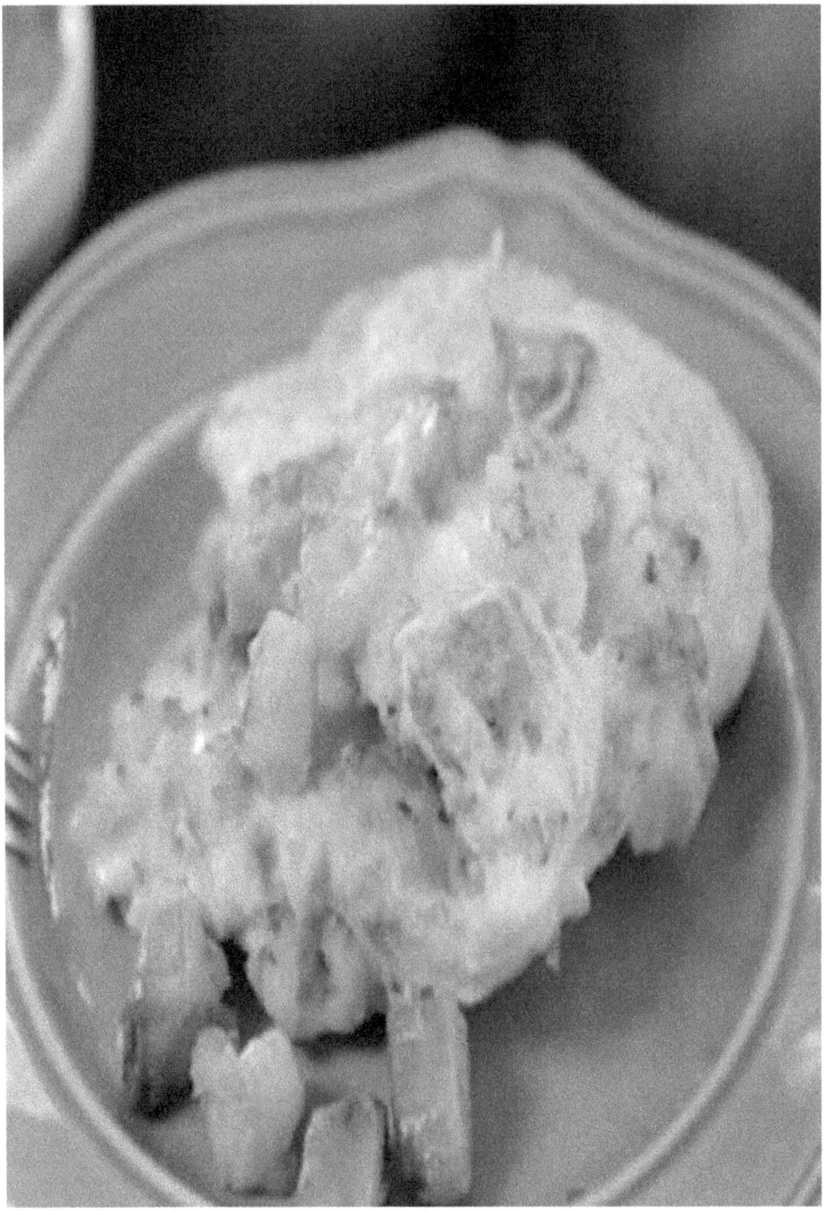

Prep Time

Total Time: 30 minutes Serves: 2

Ingredients:

¼ pounds' shrimp peeled and de-veined 1 medium tomato, diced

½ medium avocado, diced

1 tbsp. cilantro, fresh chopped

¼ tsp. sea salt

1/8 tsp. black pepper, fresh ground 1 tsp. coconut oil

4 large eggs, beaten

Directions:

1. Cook shrimp over medium heat until pink. Chop and set aside.
2. Toss tomato, avocado, and cilantro together in a small bowl. Season to taste with sea salt and black pepper. Set aside.
3. Beat eggs in a separate small bowl.
4. Heat a non-stick skillet over medium-high heat. Add coconut oil.
5. Pour half of the eggs into the hot skillet, tilting the pan gently to cover the bottom with egg. Tilt pan and lift edges of omelet to allow uncooked egg to spread to the hot part of the pan.
6. When eggs are almost fully firm, add shrimp pieces onto one half of the egg.
7. Fold omelet in half and cook for a minute more.
8. Top with tomato and avocado mixture.
9. Repeat for second omelet.

Chorizo Scrambled Eggs

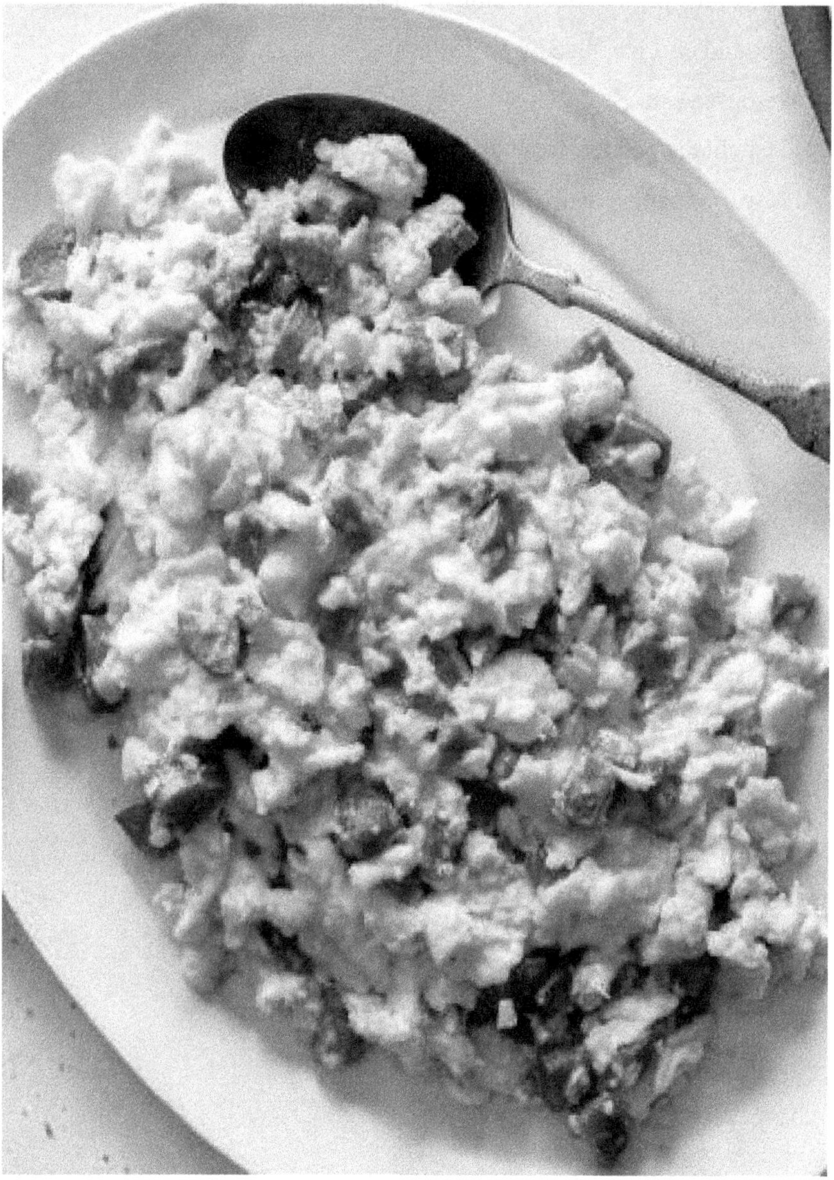

Prep Time

Total Time: 15 minutes Serves: 2

Ingredients:

1 tbsp. coconut oil

½ medium yellow diced onions 1 medium bell pepper, red diced

½ pound chorizo sliced 4 large eggs

¼ tsp. sea salt

¼ tsp. black pepper, fresh ground

¼ tsp. hot pepper sauce

Directions:

1. Heat a medium sauté pan over medium-high heat. When hot, add coconut oil and sauté onions for 5 minutes
2. Add red pepper and chorizo until the chorizo gets crispy around the edges and the onion turns slightly translucent.
3. Meanwhile, beat the eggs in a small bowl and add sea salt and black pepper.
4. Pour the eggs into the pan with the onions, pepper, and chorizo
5. Scramble the eggs softly until cooked
6. Top with hot sauce.

Egg, Bacon & Sweet Potato Salad

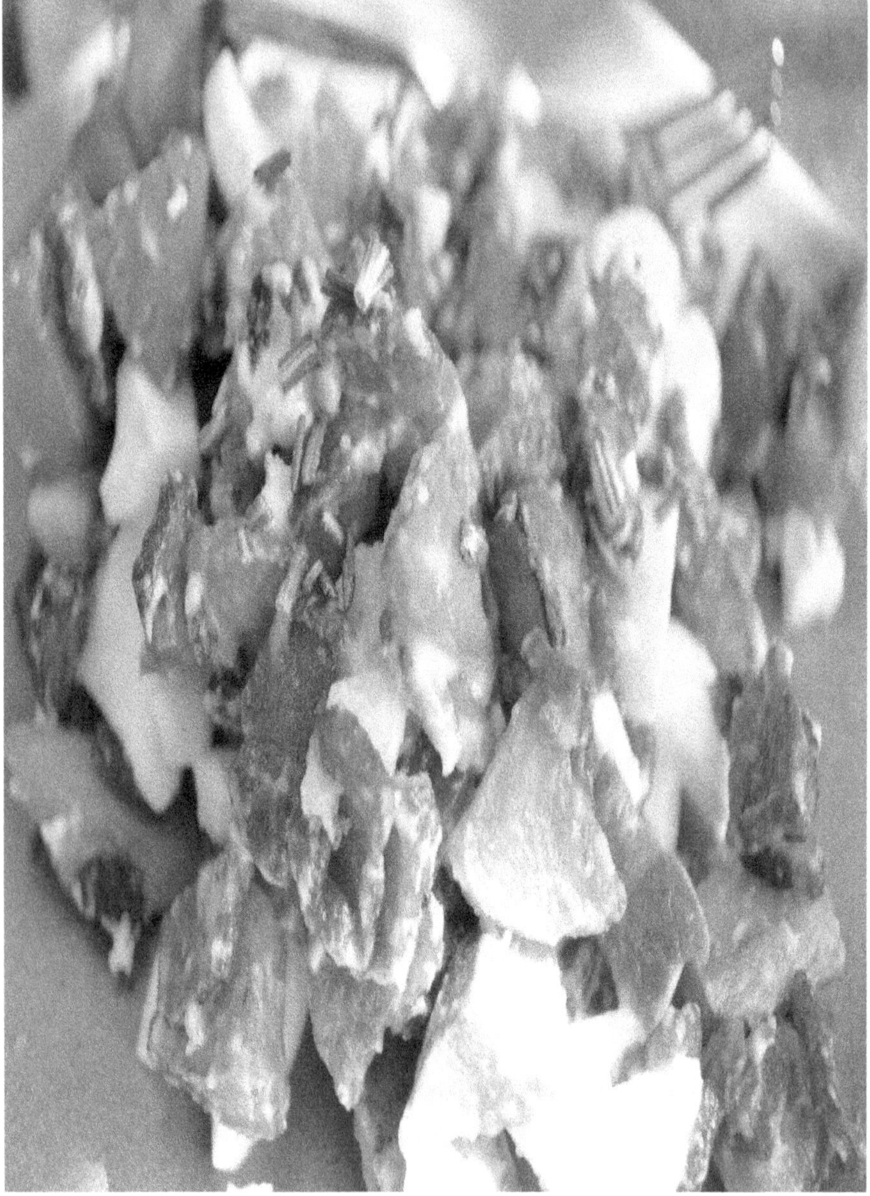

Prep Time

Total Time: 35 minutes Serves: 2

Ingredients:

1 medium sweet potato diced 2 large eggs

8 slices bacon, diced

4 tbsp. dill, freshly finely chopped 2 tbsps. paleo mayo

2 tbsps. Lemon juice

Directions:

1. Place eggs in small sauce pan, cover with cold water, cover pan and place over high heat until just before boiling.
2. Remove from heat and let sit, covered, for 13 minutes.
3. Immediately rinse in cold water, peel eggs, dice and set aside.
4. Meanwhile, dice sweet potato.
5. Heat skillet over medium-high. When hot, add bacon and cook for 5 minutes.
6. Add diced sweet potato and continue to cook until potato is tender and bacon is fully cooked.
7. In a small bowl, mix dill, mayonnaise and lemon juice.
8. Add eggs, sweet potato and bacon, and mix. Serve warm or cold.

Sausage & Roasted Pepper Omelet

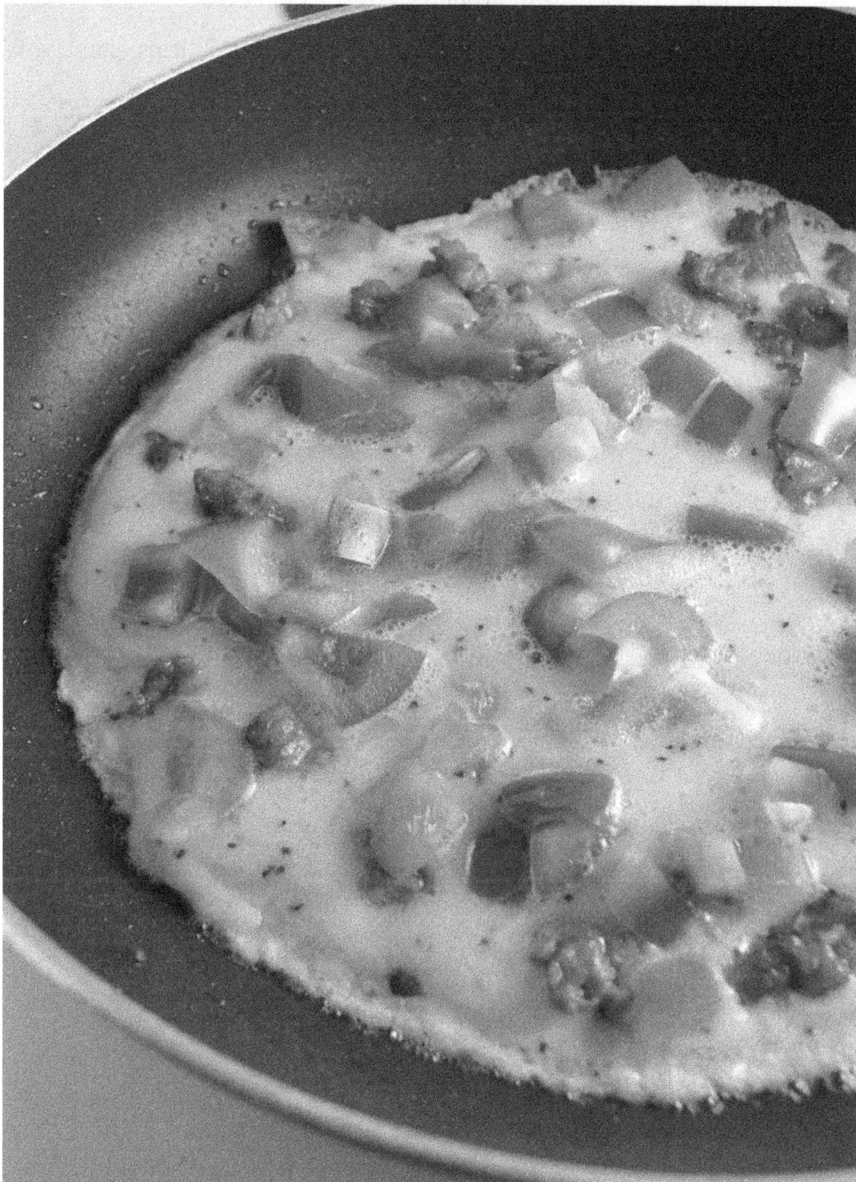

Prep Time

Total Time: 30 minutes Serves: 2

Ingredients:

1 medium poblano pepper 4 large eggs

¼ tsp. black pepper, fresh ground 2 tsp. coconut oil

½ pound Italian sausage or beef, cooked and sliced 2 tbsps. parsley, fresh chopped.

Directions:

1. Put pepper in a heavy bottomed pan over high heat. Turn pepper as skin begins to black and blister on each side. When blistered on all sides, remove from pan and put in a plastic bag with a few drops of water; seal the bag immediately with plenty of air trapped inside. Wait 5 minutes. Remove from bag, cut out seeds, remove skin and dice.
2. Meanwhile, beat eggs in a small bowl and add freshly ground black pepper.
3. Heat medium non-stick skillet over medium heat. Add 1 tsp. coconut oil when hot.
4. Add half of the egg mixture to hot pan. As the egg starts to set, add half of the remaining ingredients to one half of the pan.
5. When fully set, fold half of the egg over the filling, and cook a minute more.
6. Repeat with second omelet.

Eggs Salsa & Avocado

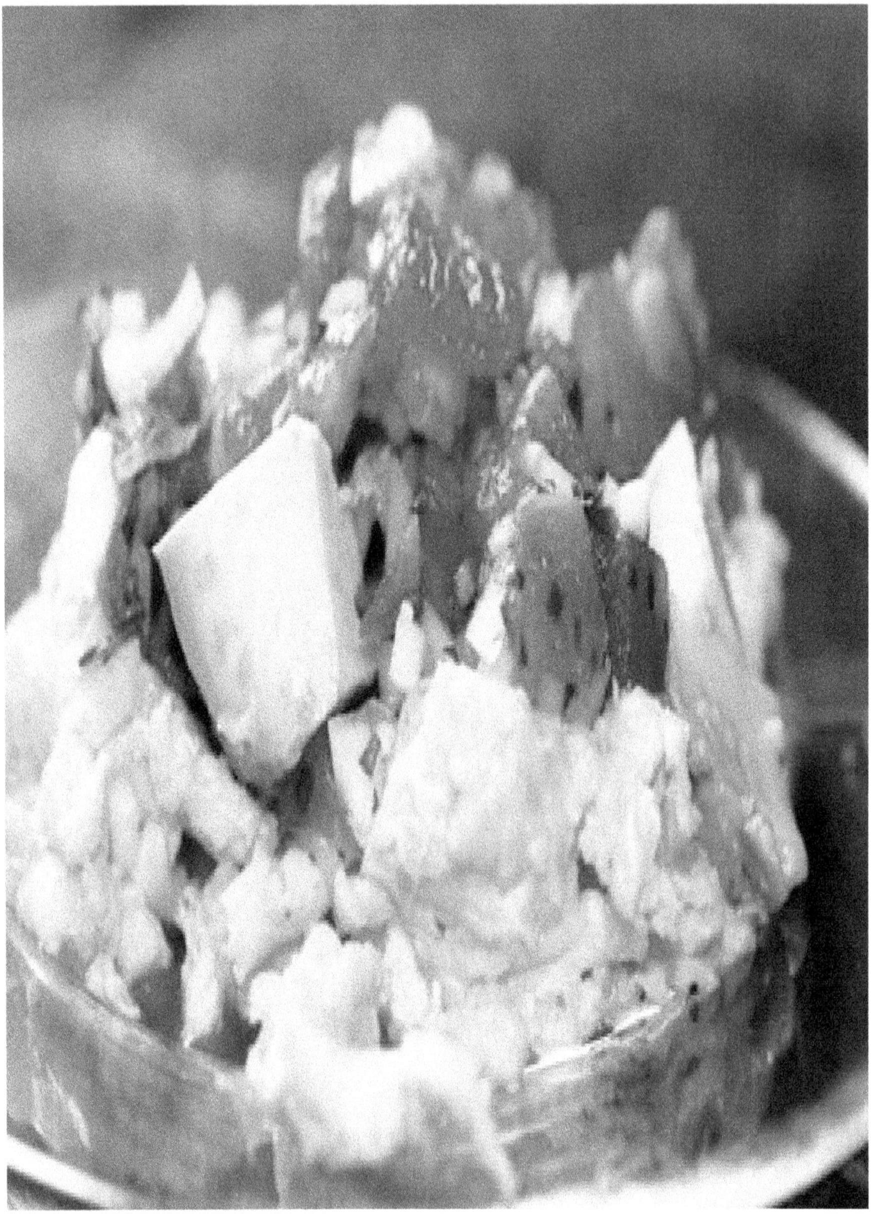

Prep Time

Total Time: 10 minutes Serves: 2

Ingredients:

4 large eggs

½ medium avocado sliced

½ cup almonds sliced or slivered 4 tbsp. salsa

Directions:

1. Heat non-stick skillet over medium-high heat.
2. Beat eggs in a small bowl, and pour into skillet.
3. Cook for 1 minute and turn heat to medium-low. Finish cooking (about 2-4 minutes longer).
4. Top with almonds, avocado and salsa. Season with freshly ground black pepper and sea salt, if desired.

Turkey Quiche

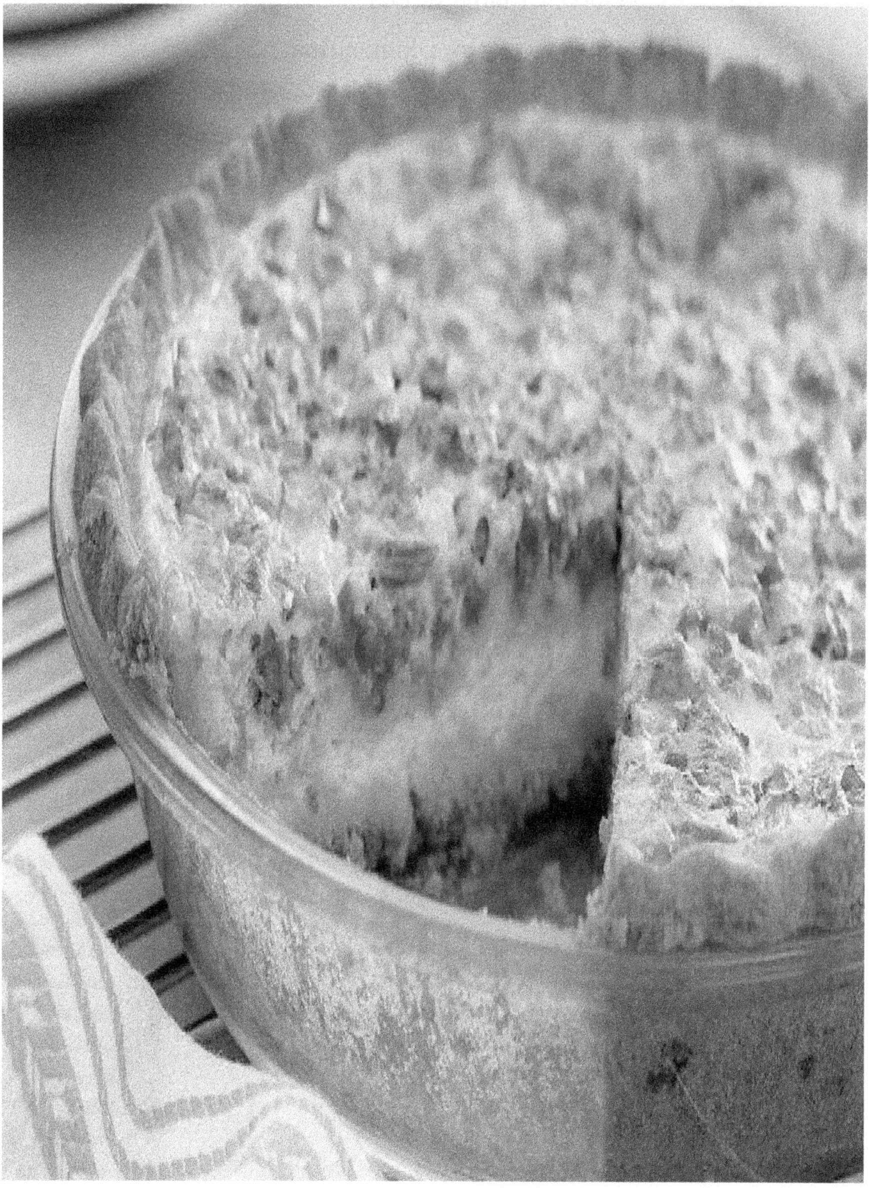

Prep Time

Total Time: 60 minutes Serves: 4

Ingredients:

8 large eggs

½ pound ground turkey 1 large shredded carrot

1 medium chopped onion 1 tsp. Dijon mustard

¼ tsp. cumin

¼ cup fresh chopped basil

¼ cup water

½ tsp. sea salt

½ tsp. black pepper 1 tbsp. coconut oil

Directions:

1. Pre-heat oven to 350 F.
2. Grease a 9-inch pie plate or 9 inch baking dish with coconut oil or bacon fat and set aside.
3. Brown the ground turkey, onions, carrots, Dijon mustard
4. And cumin together in a pan.
5. Set the turkey mixture aside to cool slightly and whisk eggs together in a bowl
6. Add fresh or dried herbs, salt, pepper, water and cooled turkey mixture to the eggs and whisk everything together.
7. Pour entire mixture into the prepared pie plate or baking dish and cook for 40 to 45 minute until set.

Almond Pancakes

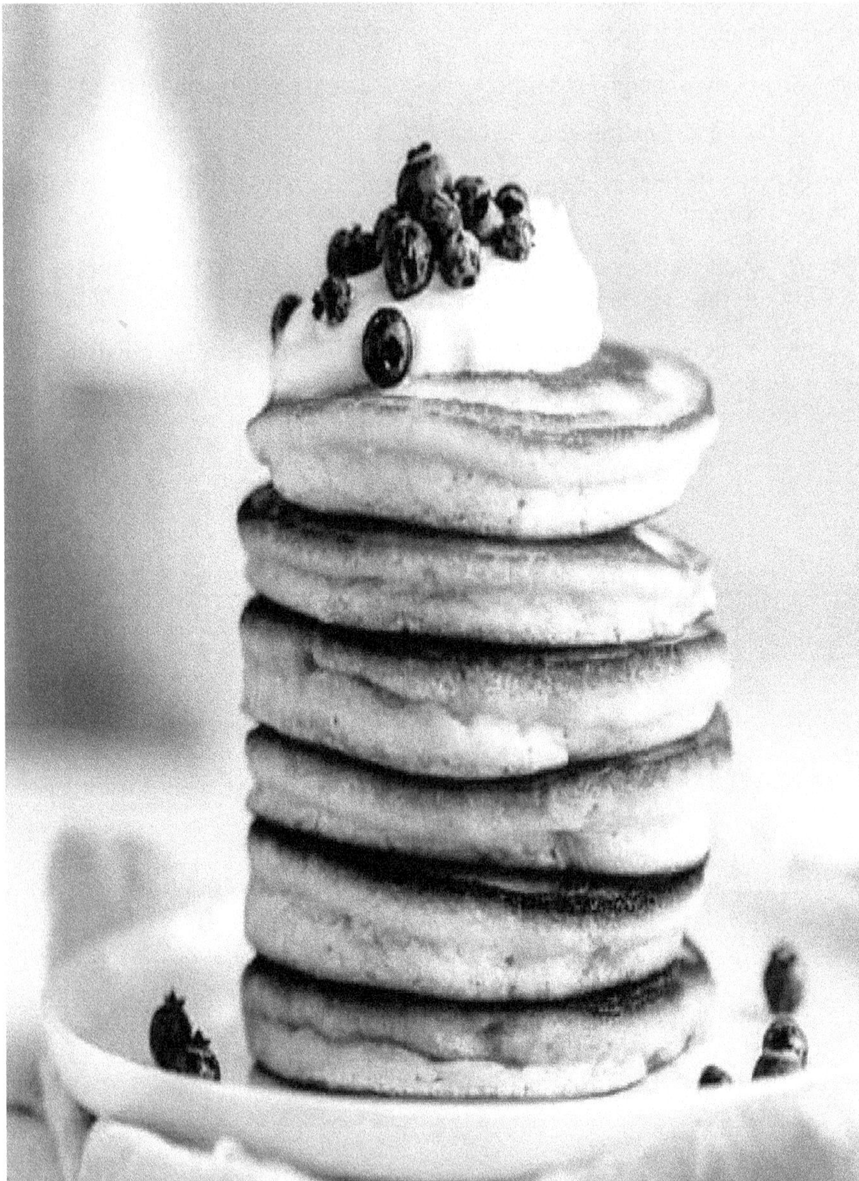

Prep Time

Total Time: 30 minutes Serves: 2

Ingredients:

1 cup almond flour

½ cup unsweetened applesauce 1 tbsp. coconut flour

2 large eggs

¼ cup water

¼ tsp nutmeg, fresh

¼ tsp. sea salt

1 tbsp. coconut oil

½ cup fresh berries

Directions:

1. Combine almond flour, applesauce, coconut flour, eggs, water, nutmeg and sea salt in a bowl, and mix together completely with a fork. The batter will appear a little thicker than normal mix.
2. Heat a non-stick frying pan over medium-low heat with coconut oil.
3. Drop 1/4 cup of batter onto the pan once it is fully heated. Spread out batter slightly if desired.
4. Flip like a normal pancake when the bubbles start showing up on the top, and cook for another minute or two.
5. Add more oil to the pan and repeat with remaining batter.
6. Top with fresh berries.

Sweet Potato Hash & Fried Eggs

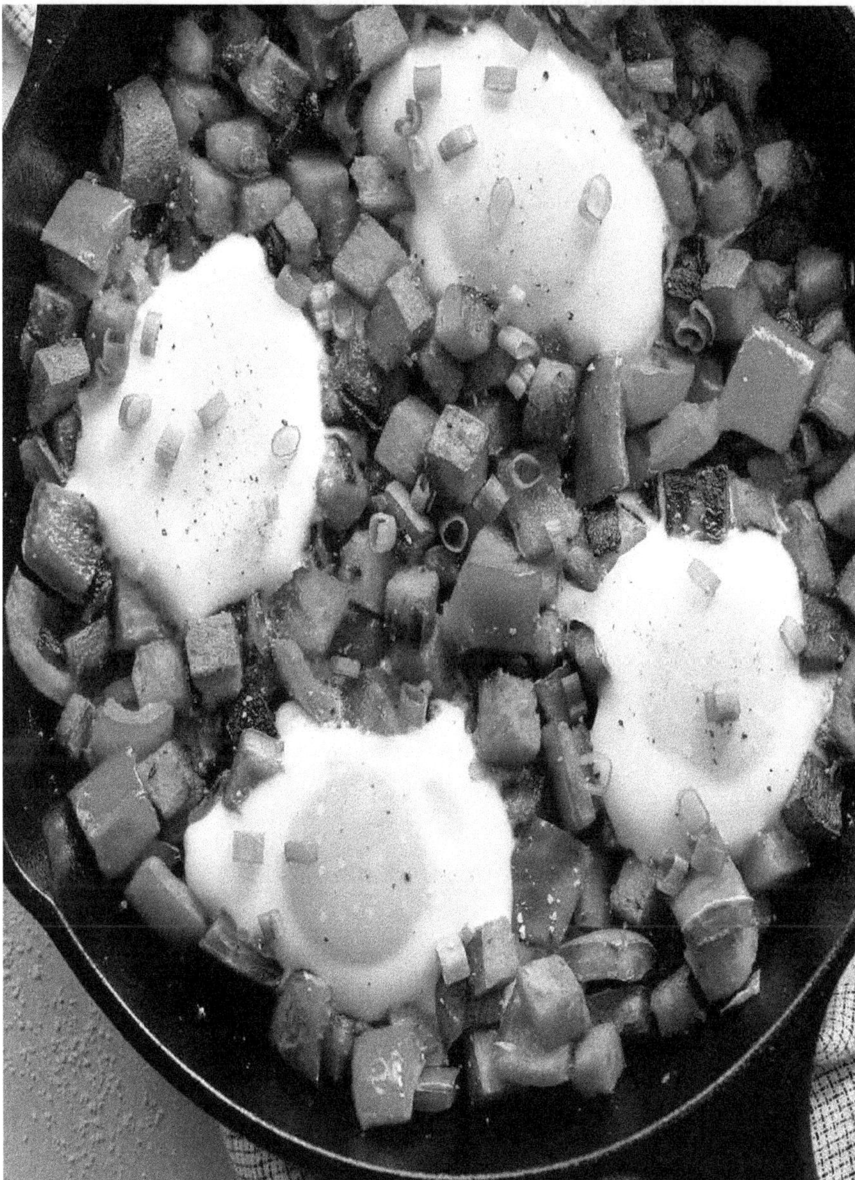

Prep Time

Total Time: 35 minutes Serves: 2

Ingredients:

1 tbsp. coconut oil divided

1 medium sweet potato, diced into ½ inch cubes

½ medium diced onion 2 medium sliced sausage

1 medium diced bell pepper 2 tbsp. water

4 large eggs

¼ tsp. fresh ground black pepper

Directions:

1. In a large skillet, heat coconut oil over medium heat.
2. Add the onions and sweet potatoes, and sauté for 5 minutes.
3. Add the sausages and continue to cook until sausages are browned and sweet potatoes are slightly softened.
4. Add bell peppers and water.
5. Cover and cook for 15 minutes or until the potatoes are completely soft, stirring frequently.
6. Meanwhile, fry eggs in coconut oil.
7. Season eggs with fresh ground black pepper and serve over sweet potato hash.

Pacific Omelet

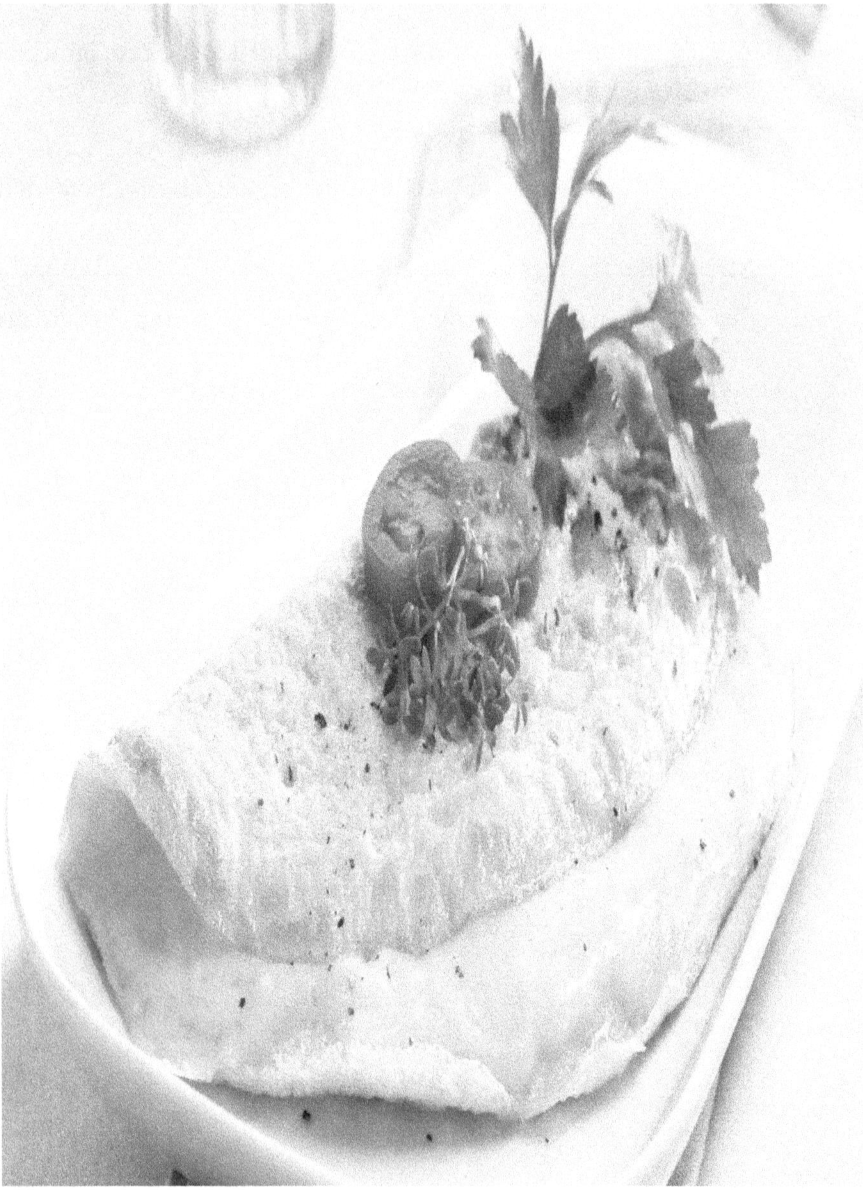

Prep Time

Total Time: 25 minutes Serves: 2

Ingredients:

4 large eggs

1 tsp. coconut oil

½ medium diced yellow onion 1 medium diced bell pepper

1 medium diced tomato 1 cup spinach

¼ pound cooked and diced ham

¼ tsp sea salt to taste

¼ tsp fresh ground black pepper

Directions:

1. Wash and chop vegetables. Set aside
2. Crack eggs into a small bowl and beat well. Set aside.
3. Heat non-stick skillet over medium heat. When hot, add coconut oil to pan.
4. Pour half of the beaten eggs into the skillet and coat bottom of the pan. When the egg has partially set, scrape the edges and tip the pan so that the uncooked egg at the top can spread to the hot cooking surface of the skillet.
5. Immediately after, add half of the vegetables and ham to one half of the omelet and continue to cook until the egg is almost fully set.
6. Using a spatula, fold the empty half over the top of the ham and veggies. Cook for 2 minutes longer, then serve.
7. Repeat the process with the remaining ingredient to make the second omelet.

Stir-Fry Sausage

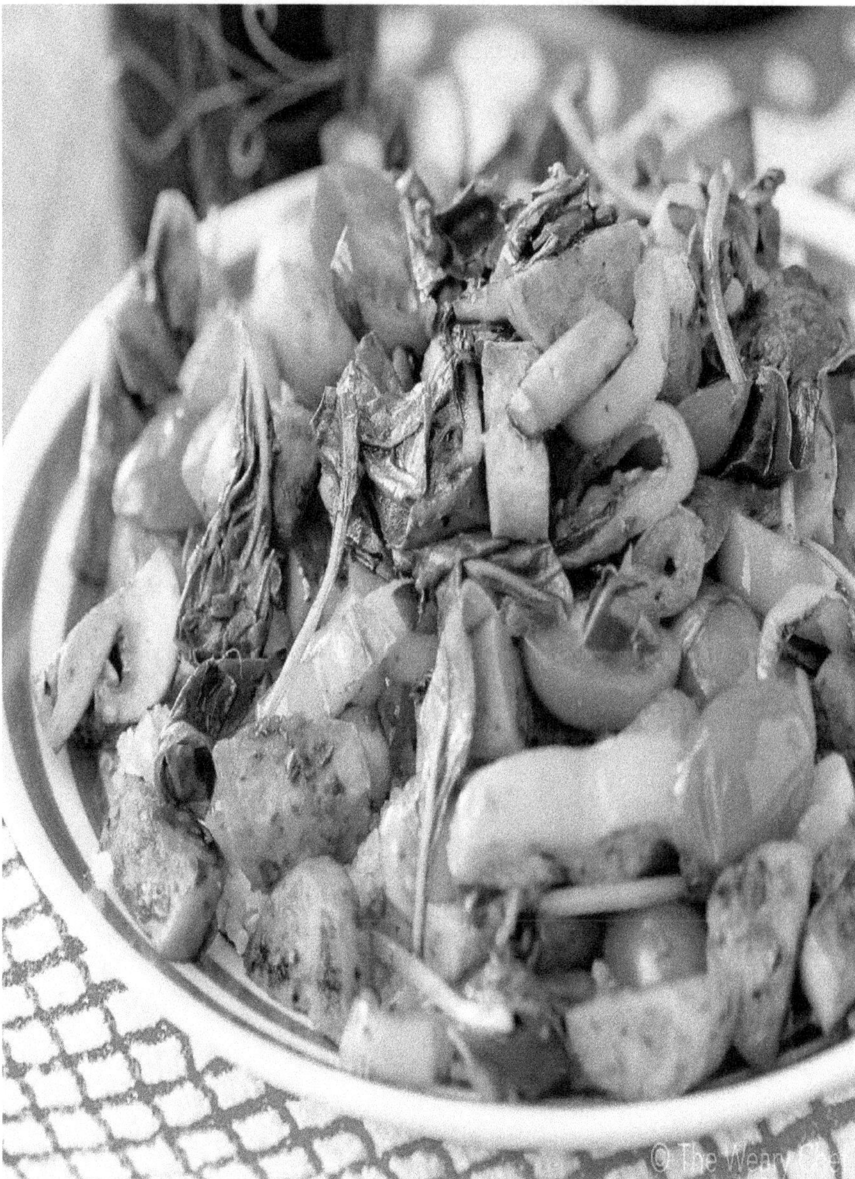

Prep Time

Total Time: 20 minutes Serves: 2

Ingredients:

1 tsp. coconut oil

½ medium diced yellow onion

½ pound sliced Italian sausage 4 cups spinach

Directions:

1. Heat a skillet over medium heat, and add coconut oil when hot.
2. Add diced onions and sauté until translucent.
3. Add sausage and cook until browned, tossing frequently.
4. Add greens, reduce heat to medium-low, and cover.
5. Serve when the greens are wilted and soft.

Cinnamon Fruit Salad

Prep Time

Total Time: 15 minutes Serves: 2

Ingredients:

1 medium peeled and diced orange 1 medium diced apple

½ cup chopped walnuts

½ tsp cinnamon

Directions:

1. Place the fruit into bowls.
2. Sprinkle with chopped nuts and cinnamon.

Pumpkin Crumb Muffins

Prep Time

Total Time: 40 minutes Serves: 4

Ingredients:

Muffins:

5 large eggs

1/3 cup canned pumpkin puree 1/3 cup coconut sugar

¼ cup coconut flour 1/8 tsp. sea salt

½ tsp. baking soda

1 tbsp. pumpkin pie spice Topping:

1/3 cup palm shortening 1/3 cup coconut sugar

2 tbsp. coconut flour

2 tbsp. ground cinnamon

Directions:

1. In a food processor, combine eggs, pumpkin, and coconut sugar.
2. Pulse in coconut flour, salt baking soda, and pumpkin pie spice until well combined.
3. Divide batter between 8 paper lined muffin cups.
4. Rinse out food processor.
5. In a food processor, combine shortening and coconut sugar.
6. Pulse in coconut flour and cinnamon.
7. Sprinkle topping over cupcake batter.
8. Bake at 350 F for 20-25 minutes.
9. Cool 1 hour.

Cranberry Walnut Scones

Prep Time

Total Time: 30 minutes Serves: 4

Ingredients:

2 cups blanched almond flour

½ tsp. baking soda 1 large egg

2 tbsp. coconut sugar 1 tbsp. orange zest

½ cup dried cranberries

½ cup walnuts chopped

Directions:

1. In a food processor pulse together almond flour and baking soda.
2. Pulse in egg, coconut sugar, and orange zest.
3. Stir in cranberries and walnuts by hand.
4. Transfer dough to a parchment paper lined baking sheet.
5. Form dough into a large circle, 1- 1 ½ inches thick.
6. Cut Dough like a pizza, into 8 slices.
7. Using a metal baking spatula move slices apart, leaving 2 inches between.
8. Bake at 350 F for 12-16 minutes until edges are browned.

Cinnamon Coffee Crumbs

Prep Time

Total Time: 50 minutes Serves: 4

Ingredients:

Cake:

2 ½ cups blanched almond flour

¼ tsp. sea salt

½ tsp baking soda

¼ cup coconut oil

½ cup honey 3 large eggs

Topping:

¼ cup coconut oil, melted

¼ cup coconut sugar

2 tbsp. ground cinnamon

½ cup sliced almonds

Directions:

1. Grease a 9 inch round cake pan with coconut oil and dust with almond flour.
2. In a food processor, combine almond flour, salt, and baking soda.
3. Pulse in coconut oil, honey, and eggs.
4. Spread the batter into prepared baking dish.
5. To make the topping, combine coconut oil, coconut sugar, cinnamon, and sliced almonds in a small bowl.
6. Sprinkle topping over cake batter.
7. Bake at 350 F for 30 minutes.
8. Cool and serve.

Orange Poppy Scones

Prep Time

Total Time: 75 minutes Serves: 6 scones

Ingredients:

2 cups blanched almond flour

¼ tsp. sea salt

¼ tsp. baking soda

¼ cup honey 1 large egg

1 tbsp. orange zest 1 tbsp. poppy seeds

Directions:

1. In a food processor combine almond flour, salt, and baking soda.
2. Pulse in honey, eggs, and orange zest.
3. Very briefly pulse in poppy seeds.
4. Roll out dough to ½ inch thick between 2 pieces of parchment paper.
5. Chill dough in freezer for 15 minutes.
6. Using a cookie cutter, cut hearts out of dough.
7. Transfer to a parchment lined baking sheet.
8. Bake at 350 F for 25-30 minutes.
9. Cool for 30 minutes.

Crepes

Prep Time

Total Time: 20 minutes Serves: 6 crepes

Ingredients:

2 tbsp. coconut flour 4 large eggs

1 tbsp. coconut oil, melted over very low heat

½ cup water

2 tbsp. coconut oil, for cooking

Directions:

1. In a food processor, pulse together coconut flour and eggs.
2. Add 1 tbsp. of coconut oil and water and pulse until thoroughly combined.
3. Heat 1 tsp. of the coconut oil in an 8 inch frying pan over medium- low heat.
4. Scoop ¼ cup of the batter onto the skillet to spread the batter to the edges of the pan.
5. Cook until small bubbles form and burst on the surface of the crepe, then flip and cook the other side, 4-5 minutes' total.
6. Transfer the crepe to a plate.
7. Repeat the process with the remaining oil and batter, then serve.

Pumpkin Cranberry Granola

Prep Time

Total Time: Overnight + 10 hours Serves: 4

Ingredients:

1 cup almonds

1 cup macadamia nuts 1 cup pumpkin seeds

1 cup roasted pumpkin or canned pumpkin puree 2-4 tbsp. honey

1 tbsp. ground cinnamon

¼ tsp. sea salt

½ cup dried cranberries, juice

Directions:

1. Place nuts and seeds in a large bowl.
2. Cover with water and soak overnight.
3. Drain and rinse the nuts and seeds, discarding soaking water.
4. Pulse nuts and seeds in food processor.
5. Pulse until coarsely chopped almost to the consistency of granola.
6. Very briefly pulse in pumpkin puree, honey, cinnamon, and salt.
7. Spread mixture onto 2 baking sheets.
8. Bake at 170 F for 10 hours, then leave in oven with temperature off, but light on, until crispy.
9. Remove from oven and stir in dried cranberries.
10. Serve with almond milk.

Orange Biscuits with Cranberry

Prep Time

Total Time: 40 minutes Serves: 6 biscuits

Ingredients:

¼ cup coconut flour

¼ tsp. sea salt

¼ tsp. baking soda

¼ cup palm shortening

¼ cup coconut sugar 3 large eggs

1 tbsp. orange zest

½ cup dried cranberries

Directions:

1. Place coconut flour, salt, and baking soda in a food processor.
2. Pulse in shortening, coconut sugar, eggs, and orange zest.
3. Remove blade from processor and stir in cranberries by hand.
4. Fill a ¼ cup scoop with patter.
5. Release batter onto a parchment paper lined baking sheet.
6. Bake at 350 F for 20 minutes.
7. Cool for 15 minutes. Serve.

Chocolate Chip Banana Pancakes

Prep Time

Total Time: 30 minutes Serves: 2

Ingredients:

1 cup raw cashews

½ tsp. baking soda 2 large eggs

½ cup mashed banana 1 tbsp. vanilla extract

¼ cup chocolate chips coconut oil for cooking

Directions:

1. In a food processor, pulse cashews until finely ground.
2. Pulse in baking soda, then pulse in eggs, banana, and vanilla until very smooth.
3. Stir in chocolate by hand.
4. Heat oil in skillet over medium heat.
5. Spoon batter 1 tbsp. at a time onto skillet.
6. Flip pancakes when bubbles form.
7. Cook for about a minute on second side
8. Serve with maple syrup.

Lemon Poppy Seed Muffins

Prep Time

Total Time: 90 minutes Serves: 20 mini-muffins

Ingredients:

¼ cup coconut flour

¼ tsp. sea salt

¼ tsp. baking soda 3 large eggs

¼ cup honey

¼ cup palm shortening 1 tbsp. lemon zest

1 tbsp. poppy seeds

Directions:

1. In a food processor, pulse together coconut flour, salt, and baking soda.
2. Pulse in eggs, honey, shortening, lemon zest, and poppy seeds.
3. Spoon batter 1 tbsp. at a time into a mini muffin pan with mini muffin liners.
4. Bake at 350 F for 8-12 minutes.
5. Cool for 1 hour and serve.

Autumn Breakfast Bars

Prep Time

Total Time: 30 minutes Serves: 8

Ingredients:

1 cup blanched almond flour

¼ tsp. sea salt

¼ cup coconut oil 2 tbsp. honey

1 tbsp. water

1 tsp. vanilla extract

½ cup unsweetened shredded coconut

½ cup pumpkin seeds

½ cup sunflower seeds

¼ cup blanched slivered almonds

¼ cup raisins

Directions:

1. In a food processor combine almond flour and salt.
2. Pulse in coconut oil, honey, water and vanilla until combined.
3. Pulse in coconut, pumpkin seeds, almond slivers and raisins until combined.
4. Press dough into an 8x8 baking dish, wetting your hands with water to pat dough down.
5. Bake at 350 F for 2 hours, then serve.

Chocolate Chip Scones

Prep Time

Total Time: 25 minutes Serves: 6-8 scones

Ingredients:

½ cup coconut flour

¼ tsp. sea salt

¼ tsp. baking soda

¼ cup palm shortening

¼ cup honey 4 large eggs

½ cup chocolate chips

Directions:

1. In a food processor, combine coconut flour, salt and baking soda.
2. Pulse in shortening, honey and eggs.
3. Stir in chopped chocolate by hand.
4. Scoop batter onto a parchment paper lined baking sheet.
5. Bake at 350 F for 12 minutes.
6. Cool and Serve.

Porridge

Prep Time

Total Time: 10 minutes Serves: 2

Ingredients:

2 tbsp. unsweetened shredded coconut 1 tbsp. pumpkin seeds

1 tbsp. brown flaxseed 1 tbsp. chia seeds

¼ cup walnuts

1 tsp. ground cinnamon

¼ tsp. sea salt

1 cup boiling water

Directions:

1. Combine dry ingredients in a food processor and blend until finely ground.
2. Pour boiling water into processor, cover with lid.
3. Blend very carefully starting on low setting the moving to high until porridge is smooth.
4. Transfer porridge to a bowl.
5. Garnish with raisins, sunflower seeds, or shredded coconut.
6. Serve.

Banana Walnut Muffins

Prep Time

Total Time: 35 minutes Serves: 5

Ingredients:

3 large eggs

¼ cup coconut oil 2 medium bananas

3 dates (remove pits)

10 drops natural sweetener

¼ cup coconut flour

¼ tsp. sea salt

½ tsp. baking soda

½ cup walnuts, toasted and chopped

Directions:

1. Place eggs, oil, bananas, dates and sweetener in a food processor; blend on medium speed until combined.
2. Add in coconut flour, salt and baking soda and blend until smooth.
3. Fold in walnuts.
4. Scoop ¼ cup batter into a lined muffin pan.
5. Bake at 350 F for 25 minutes.
6. Cool and serve.

Green Eggs

Prep Time

Total Time: 15 minutes Serves: 2

Ingredients:

4 large eggs

4 leaves large kale pinch of sea salt oil of your choice

Directions:

1. Place eggs, kale and salt in a food processor.
2. Blend on high until it is smooth.
3. Heat oil in 8 inch frying pan over medium heat.
4. Pour egg mixture in pan.
5. Cook eggs to your preferred doneness
6. Serve.

Muesli Scones

Prep Time

Total Time: 35 minutes Serves: 3

Ingredients:

2 cups blanched almond flour

½ tsp. sea salt

½ tsp baking soda

¼ cup dried cranberries

¼ cup dried apricots, cut into ¼ inch pieces

¼ cup sunflower seeds

¼ cup raw sesame seeds

¼ cup pistachios, coarsely chopped 1 large egg

2 tbsp. honey

Directions:

1. In a large bowl, combine almond flour, salt and soda.
2. Stir in dried fruit, seeds and nuts.
3. In a small bowl combine egg and honey
4. Stir wet ingredients into dry.
5. Use your hands to form dough.
6. Shape dough into 6x6 inch squares about half and inch thick.
7. Cut dough into 16 squares.
8. Bake at 350 F on parchment paper lined baking sheet for 10-12 minutes.
9. Serve.

Orange Choco Scones

Prep Time

Total Time: 30 minutes Serves: 4

Ingredients:

2 cups blanched almond flour

¾ tsp. baking soda

½ cup chocolate hips 1 tbsp. orange zest

1 large egg

3 tbsp. honey

Directions:

1. In a large bowl, combine almond flour, baking soda, dark chocolate, and zest.
2. In a smaller bowl, combine egg and honey.
3. Mix wet ingredients into dry, thoroughly.
4. Form dough into a circle that is about ½ inch thick.
5. Cut dough like a pizza, into 8 slices.
6. Using a spatula, transfer to a parchment paper lined baking sheet.

Bake at 350 F for 10-15 minutes.

Alphabetical Index

Z

CPSIA information can be obtained
at www.ICGtesting.com
Printed in the USA
LVHW051630010621
689061LV00002B/407

9 781803 073514